Also by K. Akua Gray

Today: Wellness Manifestations

The Natural Health and Wellness Manual

Veggie Delights: Holistic Health Recipes, Eating Live for Maximum Nutrition and Wellness

Akwaaba!: Dr. Akua's Ghanaian Vegan Cuisine

Holistic Sexuality

A Practical Guide to Sexual Healing

Bojakaz Management
P O Box 921
Missouri City, Texas 77459
Copyright © 2014 by K. Akua Gray

All rights reserved. No part of this book may be reproduced in any form or by any means including electronic, mechanical or photocopying or stored in a retrieval system without permission in writing from the publisher except by a reviewer who may quote a brief passage to be included in a review.

This publication was designed to provide accurate and authoritative information in regard to the subject matters covered. It is sold with the intention to educate, inform, and empower readers to make their own decisions on health, life, and well being. If you have concerns about your physical, mental, or spiritual condition consult the appropriate professional.

Cover Design: K. Akua Gray
Cover Portrait: Joshua Kenneth Gray

Printed in the United States of America
ISBN 10: 0990408906
ISBN 13: 978-0-9904089-0-1

For Chenu
My light of love for eternity

For CW
I am grateful for the experience of sacred sex from the very beginning

TABLE OF CONTENTS

Introduction
7

Chapter 1 Moving Beyond the Norm
12

Chapter 2 The Holistic Side of Sex
28

Chapter 3 Sexual Healing
49

Chapter 4 Mental and Emotional Maintenance/Relationship Intelligence
65

Chapter 5 Establishing the Divine Family Structure
98

Chapter 6 The Next Generation
112

Chapter 7 Holistic Sexual Living
118

Introduction

Holistic sexuality is a spiritual discipline that is learned and lived with a constant flow of complete openness and honesty. It nurtures the highest quality of life that can exist between a man and a woman. Holistic sexuality is the answer to not only a blissful sex life, but also a life that is filled with free flowing energy that mends broken relationships, promotes positive thinking about coexisting in peace and if lived to the fullest, will bring forth a life that enhances a system of longevity. The essence of a healing sexual union depends on both openness and honesty. Openness meaning relating to each other with a trust that is free of fear and deceit and honesty meaning no matter the difficulty, the truth will always be told to facilitate true growth in a relationship.

It is sexual energy that empowers us with the ability to make man; therefore enabling the divine qualities of both male and female. Sexual energy exemplifies the divinity and balance of man and woman as co-creators. Sexual energy yields itself as a guide to the natural powers of human attraction. The energy that has shaped the world is sexual energy. Billions of people exist in their respective areas of the world through sexual energy. Every human has life because of sexual energy. The reason life continues to exist on earth no matter what man has gone through is because of sexual energy. It is the one power that humans have the ability to use for eternal existence.

The power of sexual energy is common knowledge for the masses that choose to indulge their minds on this level; however, what is not common knowledge is how to use this powerful energy for healing and balancing the physical, mental, emotional and spiritual aspects of life. Most people live life in a state of permanent sexual dysfunction. There is however an alternative to the primitive drive and it equates more closely to divine will.

On a physical level, holistic sexuality brings awareness to the individual and the couple of the sacredness of the body they possess. Also their quest for longevity is enriched by the proper nourishment of the energy exchanged in sex. This energy exchange directly affects the internal organs, the central nervous system and the endocrine system.

Holistic sexuality exercises the mind in two ways. First, mind is energy; it has no physical form. The mind is the constant reminder that there is always an interconnection between man and woman; this shows up as attraction and desire which can very easily lead to a sexual encounter. The underlying factor to consider in this most primitive interrelation is that people were divinely designed for each other and that designation was intended to be eternal; man for woman and woman for man. People however vibrate on different frequencies, so the levels of attraction will be based on energetic compatibility. The thought process involved in coming together brings the mind into alignment with the need to remain in constant contact with self through the body of another. Second, once the male and female connection is made, the mind then surrenders to the autonomic nervous system and goes into a state of trance. This semiconscious state is the doorway to a moment of peace and relaxation that the mind needs to facilitate calm and unity for survival.

Holistic sexuality on an emotional level strengthens the limbic system by activating a series of central nervous system responses to touch. Touch activates the endocrine system's glandular functions and releases hormones that help to bring about the mind's surrender and prepares the body for orgasm. Sex is an intensely emotional experience of sharing that enriches the ability of humans to respond positively to outer body stimuli.

The spiritual components of holistic sexuality include all of the above. When the consciousness of divine union is brought to the sexual experience, sex becomes a meditation, trance becomes a prayer, and purpose living is enriched. A couple can develop unconditional selfless service to one another and inspire the growth of the relationship. As couples grow together, their moments of internal peace turn into minutes, hours, days and years of blissful sexual expression that heals in every way.

Welcome to a new realm of sexual consciousness. Forget what you've been taught about sex if it doesn't set your mind in a state of peace. Holistic Sexuality: A Practical Guide to Sexual Healing is a truth resource for people to form new thought patterns about the benefits of sex as it relates to strengthening the spirit, reconnecting to the divine, achieving immortality through sex and creating physical enhancements and manifestation that last a lifetime.

Chapter 1

Moving Beyond the Norm

Sexual Dysfunction
The normal way of relating to one another as male and female is perpetrated through the dictates of popular culture and mass media. This constrictive and destructive way of addressing and facilitating a sexual relationship causes emotional and mental disease in the form of possessiveness, jealousy, envy, confusion, anger and uninhibited passion which produces blinding rage that result in abuse and sometimes death. The widespread imbalances in sexual energy have caused massive depression in society. People for many centuries have used sex as a weapon, a reward, an addiction, a tool to control the lives of others and as a means of escape from the realities of an imbalanced life. The majority of people in the world have never had sexual relationships that have brought total peace of mind. At some point in most people's sexual relationships, there has been doubt, trauma, abuse, dissatisfaction and the confusion caused by equating sex with love. Ask any adult if any of their sexual experiences has ever fulfilled every component of their whole nature. The answer will most likely be no. This is because most people know nothing of sex except for the mechanics and they only identify with the animalistic nature of their sexuality. Sexual abuse is also a part of the norm of sexual relationships in society today. People do not know how to respond to the natural intoxicating energy that occurs

between a male and female. When this energy is felt, it is immediately directed to the animalistic sexual instincts that society has promoted. The drive of sex exists for so many as an uncontrollable component of their human behavior. They don't consider that the natural lure of sex was designed to promote the eternal stream of physical life in the universe. It is sacred. However that drive has been the cause of misery and deprivation in the lives of so many because of the perversion that have emerged in the form of molestation, rape, recreational sex, pornography and sexual exploitation.

Popular culture facilitates many constrictions when it comes to sex. A perpetrator of this type of sexual dysfunction is religion. A few secular religions teach their followers that sex is bad and sex is wrong. Their doctrines and dogma teach that women should not have sex until they are legally bound to a man who then owns that aspect of her body. The vagina was blamed for the original "sin" that caused Man to fall from God's grace and damnation to hell was promised to those who partake in its pleasures without legal rights to it. The religions with this dogma leave people in a state of fear about their sexuality. In order to control the power of birth, the powers that be have always sought to instill fear into the lives of women who are the true controllers of birth. The tactics of rape, domestic violence, female circumcision and female castration are still used to cover up the hypocrisy that lurks behind the natural need for the pleasures of the vagina. The sacred jewel, the vulva, and the pyramid within, the womb, has taken on the suffering of time and has endured the devastating effects of the many unwarranted traumas of STD, fibroids, cysts, hysterectomy and tumors; total imbalance!

In the same breath, the penis has been hailed as the weapon of righteous conquering and this thinking has caused a great rift of separation between man and woman. Modern day society still upholds the idiosyncrasies that have made men believe that because of the penis they have rights to brutality, sexism, religious superiority, and total control over the lives of other people. However, they ignore the fact that the penis has been abused as well, through the absorption of negative energy from the facets of societal expectations and guidelines of what a man should be and how he should act based on what is between his legs. The penis, in connection with the hearts of men has been broken. These unfair societal conditionings have taken men away from the honorable balance of male and female as builders of the world. It has caused men to internally bury their needs for affection, nurturing, and truth. Most men have not allowed their sexual nature to flourish to a height of peace. The penis has also suffered in the sexual games that people play.

An additional factor that has led men to take advantage of the sexual experience is the orgasm. There has been an imbalance among men and women in the sexual encounter because of man's ability to experience an orgasm at a much faster rate than woman. Therefore the orgasmic power of the female has often been ignored. In a recent survey among female clients who sought services in a holistic health center in Accra, Ghana, 99% of them had never experienced an orgasm and 85% of them did not consistently enjoy the sexual experience with their male partner. Many were very intrigued by the description of what an orgasmic experience feels like and the different ways of using this energy for nurturing the body, mind and emotional health. Many men consider the sexual experience done once their own orgasm has been achieved and it leaves the female partner in a state of physical and emotional deprivation with the unwanted feeling of being used.

The struggle between the vagina and the penis often lead people into love-hate relationships that create a continuous cycle of sexual dissatisfaction and mistrust. Everybody wants to have sex because by the laws of nature there is no way to not have the natural urge to procreate. However, because of the baggage that comes with sexual dysfunction, people have developed all types of tactics to avoid the pain of interrelating. The sexual games people play include the hunt, divide and conquer, all in the family, secret lovers, commodity exchange, if you love me, one night only, what happens here stays here, don't ask – don't tell, the orgy, oops, and so many others. Playing and games have become the norm and it has been a source of misery for both men and women; total sexual dysfunction.

Mass media's interpretation of human sexuality has become the main source of sexual education for young people in society. The cycle continues. Sex education for the young is solely based on the physical and mechanical areas. When it comes to the emotional and mental aspects of sex, adults tell young people lies to make sex seem like some insignificant event that they should not be concerned with. Instead of teaching truth when it comes to sexual terminology, they make sex trivial by giving all things related to sex cute little names like pocket book, wee wee and pee pee. Furthermore, there is no education on the spiritual aspects of sex because the majority of adults have never been taught sexual spirituality themselves. The majority of young people who are adults of now and tomorrow are often not taught anything holistic before their first sexual encounters. Lies and constrictions form the early attitudes and ideas about sex for so many. This serves as the foundation for perpetual sexual dysfunction in adulthood which is seen in most relationships and may have been experienced in your own personal life. Take a moment to think about your own sex education as a youth. The stories of first time sexual experiences have been told millions of times. Jenny contracted herpes in her first sexual experience that only lasted 5 minutes. Brian didn't know what to do so in his nervousness his erection didn't last and he was made to feel inadequate by the more experienced girl. Betty had both pain and blood. She thought she had injured herself and resolved not to have sex again. Jacob took advantage of a younger schoolmate as a dare from his friends and felt guilty after the encounter. Jasmine had sex for the first time and ran home to tell her Mom because she didn't know that her body could feel that good in being kissed, caressed, massaged and held as Peter had done, but he was six years her senior and considered an adult. What's that, one out of five of the youth that had a good experience? However, it is a fact that the odds are even greater than that with the reality of molestation, rape, and sexual misconduct as the first experience for too many.

Sexual dysfunction is attached to so many negative behaviors in society. Possession. "You belong to me and that's it!" Jealousy. "Why are you looking at her?" Envy. "Who does she think she is?" Blinding passion is one of those behaviors that usually have the most tragic endings. NEWS FLASH: "Man kills ex-wife and four children before turning the gun on himself." These are the stories and behaviors that mass media finds necessary to promote in a high number of movies, TV shows, and commercials.

Some people can't help themselves because of the power of human nature and the innate power of the sex drive. They participate in sex based on a system of mediocrity and fulfillment of their animalistic drive. By this being their main source of sexual interactions, it often turns into sexual abuse of themselves and others. They either live in a world of shame about their sexual desires or they develop the 'I don't care' attitude that helps to cover up the pain of being unfulfilled and lonely in their sexual relationships have that no substance. They know deep within that they are causing emotional pain and mental suffering to their sexual partners, and they don't have the courage to admit they have created portals of vital energy drain for all the people involved in their negative sexual existence. One of the goals of internalizing holistic sexuality is to move beyond the societal norm of negativity to a positive holistic sexual lifestyle.

The first step would be to begin to develop behaviors that facilitate the release of sexually dysfunctional thought patterns. When something needs to be changed about your environment, it has to start with self. As you read the bullet points and the next few paragraphs take a moment to think about your own sexuality and the experiences that you have had in your youth to where you are now in your sexual relationships. Your experiences are the ways in life that you learn to grow and once we know better, it is intended that we do better.

- **Sex is not evil.**
- **Sex is not for fun and games.**
- **Sex does not show love.**
- **Sex can be an addiction.**

Sex is not evil contrary to what others may say. It is a natural part of human nature that has been programmed in people for a very specific reason; the most obvious reason is procreation.

Sex is not for fun; it is not something that should be looked at as being a toy or as something to go out and find to play with for a moment of enjoyment. These attitudes all feed into dysfunctional thought patterns.

Sex is not a game; it is not about conquer and destroy or beating the genitals up. That comes from both the sexually dysfunctional female and the sexually dysfunctional male. The law of reciprocity says that what you put out there, you get back and if a person has reached a certain level of ascension playing with sex no longer fits into their quest for the higher good.

Sex does not show love. There is an overall misconception about love being an emotion. Love is actually an energy vibration that is in complete existence in life at every moment. This understanding is sometimes hard to grasp. When a person says, "I love you", what they are really doing is validating feelings of happiness or the emotional euphoria that is felt by the body's release of hormones during intimacy. When a person says, "I don't love you anymore", they are really emotionally expressing hurt, anger, disappointments and fears. Love is not an emotion, it is universal energy. The universal energy of love is an energy of connection between everything that exists in the seen and unseen world. Love is a powerful vibration to concentrate and direct when necessary for the realignment of an individual or group with their divine purpose. In other words, we are in a complete existence of love at all times. The feel of the sun's warmth on your face is love. The sound of your mother's voice is love. The reason you can look at others with respect is love.

One other thing to be aware of in the dysfunctional thought patterns involving sex is that sex can be addictive. Sexual addictions develop from the hormonal responses in the body. During sex and orgasm the body releases endorphins that create euphoric feelings throughout the cellular system. These feelings of sexual pleasure with the release of pheromones between the sexes always have the potential of creating addictions in the spiritually weak. Using sex as a way to escape the pressures of life is a form of this type of addiction. It promotes an indiscriminate quest for a physical encounter without any consideration for the mental, emotional or spiritual well being of the person that is considered the prey. Sexual encounters are taken to heart because of religious and moral beliefs. However, the very real physical urge that can overpower that belief will also entangle believers in a web of sexual perversions they use to take advantage of others or create the risk of being taken advantage of by those who are only looking for the 'good time' to relieve their sexual frustration.

Evaluating What You Need To Change
The following list of questions is designed to help in the realization of areas in life that are directly linked to sexual behavior. It is a good exercise to meditate on these questions and speak truth to yourself concerning your answers.

Are you jealous and possessive in your relationships? Why?

Does your desire to be needed create unhealthy attachments to people who make you feel bad about yourself?

Have you been cheated on or lied to by a lover? How did you deal with moving forward?

Do you avoid being loved because of past abuse?

Do the emotional requirements of a sexual relationship frequently overwhelm you?

Do the physical requirements of a sexual relationship frequently overwhelm you?

Do you seek out opposite personalities in your sexual partners?

Has a past sexual experience made you afraid to trust?

Do you feel you have to measure up in your sexual experiences?

Do you always feel under pressure to perform sexually with new partners?

If you find yourself always in a jealous and possessive state in your relationships, this is actually a real fear spawned by the inability to internalize the knowledge that the universe is abundant. This is also a sign that there is not a solid level of appreciation and gratitude in your relationships. If there is real appreciation and gratitude in a relationship, the couple would be able to bless and send light to the things and people that your mate admires and is drawn to. Fear of losing someone and becoming angry at another because of the choices a person makes, shows a level of emotional, mental and spiritual immaturity that will be a scar and a hindrance to the relationship achieving its highest potential.

It is very difficult for people to break their emotional addictions in relationships. They often find themselves going through repeated episodes of drama that are like instant replays relationship after relationship. If the same negative things happen in two or more consecutive relationships, that is a sure sign that the responsibility of failure is not just "them", it's you also. Therefore, taking time in between relationships to work on you is critical. This in between work should include reconditioning your mental faculties from negative thinking to positive thinking. Affirmative evaluations of how you create or allow discord in communication, support, planning, achieving your goals, educating yourself of life and building an impeccable character should also be a focus in your relationship renewal growth.

If you have been hurt by relationships in your past and you find it difficult to move forward, a relationship break should be considered another opportunity to take time to recondition and heal your emotional faculties. The pain couples can put each other through in a relationship is real, however when the best practices for increasing emotional maturity are put into place with consistency, individuals and couples are able to work through emotional strains.

An emotion is a biochemical response in the body disseminated throughout the central nervous system. That is why when we feel an emotion, we feel it all over the body from head to toe. This biochemical response on a physical level only last three seconds however, these few moments in time make a mental impression that is stored in the brain's memory for recall at anytime. In the emotionally immature person, these memories are recalled and redistributed through the central nervous system as if the original emotion is happening all over again right then. This makes the person dwell in a state of negative emotional recall. Emotions pause the body, mind, and spirit for just a moment to receive and learn from outer body stimulus from the world around us. When people habitually mentally recreate past emotional states, they become crippled in their ability to move forward and sometimes subconsciously seek out others that will again produce situations that confirm their emotional addictions.

It is meant for humans to feel the full range of emotions, but it was not meant for humans to dwell in states of constant emotional upheaval. There are two important simple questions to ask yourself when you are stuck in an addictive emotional recall. First, what lesson did I learn from this situation? And two, how important is this to the progress of my purpose in life? If you learned the lesson which is usually an awareness of what to do and what not to do, then it will be easy for you to move forward. If the emotion serves no purpose in helping you with your goals in life, then it would be wise to release it in peace and keep it moving.

The mechanics of sex often have couples competing to provide sexual pleasure. The degree of possessive behavior that is involved with sexual relationships leads people to try to out perform each other or the last partner that their mate was with. This behavior puts unnecessary pressure on individuals and it takes away from the ability that sex has to elevate the conscious levels of awareness. This type of pressure would be considered mental sexual dysfunction. To release this type of behavior, a couple must function in the now and ask each other before a sexual relationship begins what they would like in the experience, that way the sexual encounter is a personally designed give and receive exchange of open communication.

The want for a better sexual relationship begins with recognizing where change is needed as an individual. Unfortunately, there are very few people who have learned at an early age about the sacredness of sex and even fewer have been properly prepared to enter into a wholesome relationship at the beginning of their adult life. However, it is never too late for change.

Chapter 2

The Holistic Side of Sex

Holistic Sexual Thought Patterns

To be whole is to first gain and accept the knowledge of your true nature; then allow yourself the freedom to express and experience life naturally. Being whole is also recognizing and releasing all fear in every situation in life. Fear separates and causes the body, mind and spirit to contract into insecurity and loneliness. Contraction denies healthy relationships and true intimacy. (Sherwood 1992) True intimacy is fearlessly opening your soul to the divine self that is reflected in the mates you choose. If they are right for you, your whole being will say "yes" and any fears from past and present conditioning will melt away. There will be no doubt. Whether this opening is permanent or not, is to be determined, however, if you are able to receive the lesson of growth from your time and experiences with the person, then the relationship was right for you at the time.

The dysfunctional sexual thought patterns are real in everyday life. There is a way to heal from the norm beginning with changing the way we think about sex. There must be a reprogramming of the senses, and the mental pictures, change also includes making peace with the lessons of past experiences and a commitment to learn and apply holistic sexual standards to all future encounters with discipline and free will.

Where are you in your sexual maturity? What is your dominant sexual faculty? A person's sexual relationships are a reflection of their overall character. People are unique in personality and life experiences which brings about preferences that makes a person's dominant sexual faculty either physical, emotional, mental or spiritual.

Honestly answer yes or no to the following questions to discover your dominant sexual faculty. Knowing where you are in your sexual maturity will help in your desire for sexual progress.

1. Immediately after sex, do you enjoy being touched and staying close to your mate?
2. Is your sex drive stronger in the evening?
3. Are you usually satisfied with one sexual encounter a night?
4. When your mate rejects or shies away from your sexual advances, are you ok with that?
5. Do you share all of your social and recreational activities with your mate?
6. Do you like prolonged sex?
7. Are you ok with public affection?
8. Do you prefer to have more than one sexual relationship at a time?
9. Is your first attraction to a potential mate their intellect?

10. Do you feel satisfied sexually if your mate has an orgasm and you don't?
11. Do you express honest emotions through sound during sex?
12. Are you honest with your mate when you do not want to have sex?
13. Is your mate more jealous and possessive than you?
14. Do you usually make up first after you and your mate have a disagreement?
15. Do you put more energy into making your relationship work than your mate?
16. Do you express your sexual creativity with your mate freely?
17. Are you ok with your mates sex drive decreasing as the relationship progresses?
18. If you found out that your mate is "cheating" would you try to work through the betrayal?
19. Is romance just as important to you as sex?
20. Did you go through a rites of passage ceremony going into adulthood?

To determine your dominant sexual faculty add up all your yes answers and use the 100% scale to calculate your score. For example if you have 12 yes answers your score would be 12 out of 20, which is 60%, Then use the following scale to determine your faculty.

10% - 25% is a physical sexuality
30% - 50% is an emotional sexuality
55% - 75% is a mental sexuality
80% - 100% is a spiritual sexuality

The physical faculty is the most basic of sexual natures, it is the animalistic drive that all people possess, however, someone with this as their dominant faculty will be highly dysfunctional in their sexual relationships. The immaturity that embodies this level of living will take an immense amount of mental effort and consistency to change to a positive sexual vibration.

The emotional faculty pinpoints a slight progression in the maturity of the sexual nature of the individual. The emotional connections between people can help sustain a level of commitment. Unfortunately, the unhealthy attachment factor also breeds negative emotions that are often suppressed or expressed as jealousy, anger, and possessiveness.

The mental faculty involves a very clear level of maturity in the physical and emotional aspects of a person's sexual nature. They are able to think beyond sexual stimulation and emotional insecurities. However, there is still a lack of wholeness in the overall sexual nature which often leads to a level of dishonesty in trying to please their mates.

The spiritual faculty is manifested in a sexual nature that supports the unconditional mode of interrelating. Someone who is dominant in this sexuality will actually be more receptive to the concepts and lifestyle of holistic sexuality because they have already developed an appreciation and sense of gratitude for this sacred energy.

A divine union sexual experience is facilitated by a spiritually based physical connection. It is the acknowledgement of the divine energy that exists between all people. It brings focus to the intimate connection of coexistence that two people share when they commit to assist each other with their purposes in life. A divine union, formerly known as marriage, facilitates the platform for consistency in mental, physical, emotional and spiritual growth of two individuals usually for an extended period of time. Spiritual ascension through sex allows one to tap into the energy patterns that regulate consciousness. The three glands in the brain that formulate the openings to these energy portals are the hypothalamus, pineal and pituitary glands. Each gland has a direct link to the physical, mental and emotional functions of human sexuality, the basis of which is the desire for spirit to manifest in the

̇al. The hormonal connection to the unseen as ̇rt of sex is often ignored on a conscious level ̇til the body reaches the orgasmic state and then ̇he name of god in all its' form is usually the first words that are uttered at that point in the sexual act, even among those who have no god.

Sex is for Healing

Imagine having an endless supply of an energy medicine that heals completely with no side effects. Sex is a generator for this type of quantum energy. Because sex activates three of the most powerful glands in the body, the release of sexual hormones has great regenerative elements for the body's natural daily cell replacement, organ realignment, cleansing functions and longevity. When the physical body feels good, it promotes the healing essence of the spiritual, mental and emotional bodies also. Sex provides a natural vortex for healing energy to be channeled.

Sex is for Immortality

Immortality is relative to individual belief and that renders it functional. Sex has created an endless flow of genetics through the bloodline of every person that has ever existed and that will ever exist. We have all lived forever. The body was designed to live for hundreds of years if life is lived in a regulated environment that supports the full holistic functions of its mechanism. The loss of the original knowledge pertaining to immortality has made life become shorter and shorter through the years. Sex is a part of the physical faculties that assists the body in obtaining the strength, drive, stamina, agility, rejuvenation, and youthfulness that is needed for long life. If one wants to stay healthy and fit, then an active sex life based on holistic thought patterns will be an asset to the goal of immortality. With a healthy sex life a person can reach set goals of longevity and the gift of procreation also facilitates one to the immortal form. That is only done through sex.

Sex is for Physical Strength
Obtaining and maintaining physical strength through sex is another benefit for the body when one aspires to holistic sexual thought patterns. Because sex is a mechanical act of human bodies, the motion that one takes into the sexual experience naturally provides the muscles, skeleton and organs a soothing "workout" that builds, tones and strengthens. In best sex practices, both man and woman should find comfortable ranges of motion that add to the experience for themselves and their partner.

Sex is for Procreation

The continuation of the world is in the reproductive system of man and woman. One of the most beautiful experiences families can have is birth. Acknowledging the presence of the divine in sex is one of the greatest gifts a couple can bring to each other. What that says is, "I know you are a divine and unique spiritual entity in my life and I honor you for who you are as the balance of the universe." Coming together for sex ignites your powerful sensual nature in its primary function in this physical realm. Sex is full of wonderful excitement in how it connects people to the ecstasy of creation. Sex is the reason why human life still exists on this planet. Without the procreation aspect of human nature, there would be no human. Each person is of special design based on genetics and the continuation of the process of procreation should be honored as supreme. The man and woman exercise their powers of god quality each time a child is conceived. The woman being the originator of human form also controls the rhythmic flow of procreation through the divine feminine vibrational alignment with the magnetism of the moon. Each month her body chemistry rises like the ocean's tide and she vibrates with an air of openness that facilities the activation of the natural desires of the man or men in her life. It is a natural hormonal draw that confirms her ability to conceive and she often unconsciously through definitive but subtle feminine action and a desire to be sexually fulfilled, says, "Let us make man".

It is meant for people to create, create, create and create. Keep in mind that humans were meant to live for hundreds, even thousands of years. When a little girl is born in her ovary sacs she is equipped with thousands of ovum. By natural design, once she reaches puberty it is scientific knowledge that she will release one ovum a month to facilitate her ability to conceive and birth children. We are now taught by modern science that the age range for a woman to be fertile is from puberty to 51. That is a total of about 30 to 40 years. If a woman releases 1 egg per month for 30 years, not counting the months of pregnancy, that would only be a total of 360 ovum. Hmmmm, but she was born with thousands? The numbers are not adding up and women have bought into the ignorance and pressure to suppress their reproductive health based on what the male dominated medical culture has said is normal for her. However, there are many reports in non-western societies that prove women are capable of conceiving and baring children well into their 60's, 70's, 80's and beyond. Otherwise why was she given thousands of eggs?

Men too have downplayed their supreme abilities in the process of procreation. Men have a renewable source of energy in their reproductive system. The sperm and semen if nurtured with correct living can facilitate the production of life well into their grand ages. However, for men, the issues are not so much societal pressures, but societal vices that cause the man's ability to procreate to dwindle at very early ages through prostate stress and impotency. How a man takes care of his body has everything to do with his sexual health and ability to procreate. Alcohol abuse, chemical medications, poor diet, excessive mental and emotional stress are all factors in a man's diminished procreative potential. Both men and women find it normal to be sexually castrated because the societal message that says you are useless after sixty years of age continues. However, if both man and woman realigned themselves with the natural rhythms of nature and divine law, they would have no issues or concerns with bringing forth life into this world for many generations.

Getting to know yourself sexually is a major requirement in living by holistic sexuality standards. Understanding first the powerful energy for healing and balancing happens through the physical, mental, emotional and spiritual aspects of your being is necessary to achieve sexual balance.

Vagina and Penis Bliss

Maryse Condé wrote, that it matters not what deformities a woman may possess, there is still some man who is willing to look beyond that misshapenness to get between her legs. The vagina is a physical passage way to the essence of the physical, mental, emotional and spiritual manifestations of what makes woman a Goddess. It is a vessel of connection intended for the divine rites of procreation. How do you see your vagina? Is it the beautiful passage way of life that it was intended to be or is it withdrawn from abuse, neglect, pain, disease, emotional stress, too much bad energy and confusion? A vagina in need of healing is one that knows suffering and disconnection from the divine, it knows nights of "you know this is not the man for you why are you allowing this to happen again" or "I am afraid to tell anyone this is happening to me" or "Why is there so much blood and pain!" Restoring your vagina back to health takes making some serious choices about what you allow your vagina to experience. This involves empowering yourself with courage to fight any vagina abuse that is still lingering from the past or that you may face in the future. Develop a regimen of vagina nurturing with eating fresh fruit, vulva cleansing and massage, appropriate monthly cycles of rest for regeneration and relaxing spa baths.

The feminine divine has a direct relationship with the moon's energy. The reproductive cycle of the woman follows the lunar calendar. The moon controls the waters of the earth, and it has a drawing force on each woman in her child bearing years. If a woman is healthy, she will find that her menstrual cycle follows the patterns of the moon. Through the course of a year if she pays close attention she will notice that her period, at certain parts of the year, will be in alignment with the new moon and as time goes on during the year, later she will notice that her cycle has eventually come in alignment with the full moon. If she is also spiritually in sync, her cycle, the new moon and the solstices will line up and her cycle, the full moon and the equinoxes will line up as well. Women have the ability to use their lunar alignment powers to affect change among the sub lunar forces if they are aware of the divinity that they possess. It is woman who dictates the natural patterns in the sexual relationship.

A woman has different vaginal moisture levels during certain times of the month. Sometimes the vaginal secretions are very thick and sometimes very wet and thin. Each month her body prepares for conception and pregnancy. The menstrual cycle (of 28 days) is generally divided into four phases, with major events occurring in each phase. The menstrual phase is what is known as the period. This may last for 3-5 days.

Right after the menstrual cycle, the woman's body goes through a regenerative phase of rebuilding called the proliferative phase when new thick endometrium is formed in the uterus. Her sex drive is at a minimum during this time and she is not usually interested in having sex or prefers mildly passionate sexual encounters that don't last long. This minimal sex drive ends at ovulation. The vaginal moisture level is at a minimum and thick. This phase is 6 to 14 days in the 28 day cycle.

The ovulatory phase is when the ovum is released from the ovary. It occurs some 14 days after the start of menstruation. The vaginal fluids increase during this phase, they become very wet, full of pheromones and the female sex drive has a natural increase. The woman is more ready, willing and able to participate in sex because her body's hormones are now dictating to her sexual glands that now is the time for procreation.

The secretory phase occurs between ovulation and the start of the period again, and lasts about 14 days. At 3 – 5 days before the menstrual cycle the woman's sex drive accelerates and her desire for sexual fulfillment becomes irresistible. The vaginal fluids are very wet, watery and plentiful during this phase. In other words, this is the body's naturally intense drive to achieve fertilization. When the woman is in sync with how her body naturally performs, she is empowered to guide her sexual experiences in a way that benefits her body's rhythm, thus her sexual health. This is the foundation of vagina bliss. Enjoy a happy vagina!

3 Day Rule
Man's reproductive glands produce sperm and semen. They are a renewable resource in the male body, and as a renewable resource, it takes time for the body to regenerate the seminal fluids of the body. When a man ejaculates after not having sex for an extended period of time, the ejaculation is very potent. However, if he persists with multiple ejaculations in a short period of time, there is a significant decrease in the amount of semen and sperm that is released. The intense feeling of orgasm is still present with ejaculation, however, some men have admitted to experiencing pain when the reproductive fluids have been drained in such a manner. In holistic sexuality, men are taught to preserve their vitality with the 3 Day Rule. Which simply says, wait three days between ejaculations to allow the body enough time to regenerate the vital sexual fluids. When I first introduced this concept, men found it amusing and beyond their scope of

understanding in their present frame of mind. However, with such as references Mantak Chia's, Taoist Secrets of Love: Cultivating the Male Sexual Energy, and Sacred Sexuality Ancient Egyptian Tantric Yoga, by Muata Ashby to solidify this rule. It is for those who are serious about their sexual health and can internalize the need for self-preservation and orgasm retention. Following the 3 Day Rule does not mean a man should not have sex for three days after each ejaculation; it means that he should not ejaculate even if he does have sex by practicing semen retention. Semen retention requires that in the motion of sex when the male reaches the point where ejaculation is about to happen, instead of allowing the semen to flow forth from the penis, the male stops movement and the ejaculation by concentrating his mind on allowing the sexual vibration that has built up to slowly dissipate with an internal ejaculation which provides a very similar feeling to the external ejaculation. Orgasm retention provides the man's body with a very high nutritional and energetic boost. This technique is used throughout many facets of holistic sexuality; it would be a good technique for men to develop for their holistic health and to enjoy penis bliss!

Divine Reflection

Is your mate your *"divine reflection"*? In coining this aspect of reference to those we share our lives with, in the capacity of mating, partnering and procreating, my intentions is to affect thought pattern changes for a deeper self awareness. When you think of something as divine, you give it god essence, divine energy, and when you think of a reflection, you give it the quality, quantity and value of self. Therefore, your divine reflection is the oneness of the divine energy that you are. It is good to do some self checking when it comes to using this kind of terminology, because if you are selfish, jealous, possessive and in alignment with the norms of sexuality of this society, then it is very likely that person standing on the other side of you in the form of your mate is a reflection of what you are at this point in your life. If you are dysfunctional, then nine times out of ten you have someone dysfunctional standing on the other side of you saying, "I love you". If you are working on yourself and healing from the dysfunctional ways of society, then again nine times out of ten if you invite a mate into your life at that time, they are probably at that same level of seeking and working on themselves as well. There is a quality control assessment that you can use in receiving a mate of your standards that I recommend.

Make a list of ten or more things that you would like to have in a mate that would be ideal and in alignment with your soul's peace. After you complete this list, take some time to review it to make sure that YOU ARE THE LIST. In other words you must become the list because you attract what you are. This is a good assessment to do for yourself at any stage of your relationship because we are forever changing and growing as individuals. Humans have vibration frequencies that are a part of how we interact with each other. It is the law of nature that those on similar frequencies will be attracted to one another. You cannot expect someone who has achieved enlightenment to lower their vibration, nor can you expect that someone on a low vibration to be able to automatically vibe with you because you know that you can teach them how to be what you want them to be, that's going to be a very frustrating journey.

In our relationships, most of us have learned that people are in our lives for a reason or a season. You don't own anyone and no one owns you. People have free will and there are times when relationship seasons end with certain people, and to that we say, it's ok to let go and move forward to what is next in your development for your greatest good. Embracing this form of detachment is what we holistically call, an attitude of gratitude. You are able to honor your mate for the time they spent with you adding enrichment to your life and assisting you with lessons of progress and ascension for what is coming next. Relationships are the building blocks for achieving your highest good.

Changing our thought patterns about sex and relationships is the primary endeavor when one of the goals in life is holistic sexuality. There is so much more to holistic sex that makes this form of sexually relating a fascinating and healing lifestyle.

"When you reserve a special time for something, you make it sacred."

If you could choose a set time for sex, what would it be? The most popular answer has been right before sleeping at night. Good answer. Between 7pm and 9pm, is the best time for sex. Every organ in the body has an optimal functioning time throughout the course of each twenty four hours. The reproductive organs are operating at their optimal functioning level after the digestive system processes have ceased; the excretory process of the body has slowed, and before the regenerative process of the body begins at 9pm.

Ideally if there was no electricity and we didn't have all the modern machines that keep us up late at night, what would we do after dark? Right, we would go to sleep. When we sleep, the cleansing and regenerative organs are operating at their optimal functioning levels. The liver and the gall bladder cleanse the blood and help formulate and channel waste to be released through the bowels. The respiratory system sends the body automatically into deep breathing to release gaseous waste and toxins through the lungs. Once new solid waste is formed the large intestines are ready to release at the start of the morning. All of these cleansing processes take place between 9pm and 5am. This is the reason why 6 to 10 hours of sleep at night is recommended. It gives the body a chance to become whole again every day.

Having sex during the ideal functioning time of the reproductive organs, the sex glands release hormones that send the body into a state of euphoria which harmonizes and relaxes all of the organs in the body. If orgasm is achieved or orgasm retention is performed, then the body is vibrating with those feel great hormones from head to toe. This state of harmony then facilitates the energy of cleansing and regeneration of the blood, the vital organs and final assimilations of the nutrients that were taken in for the day, this is one of the reasons it is said that sex helps you stay young.

Emotional connections

The emotions are neurological and hormonal responses triggered by inner memory and outer body stimuli. People often live in their emotional selves and most of their emotional response to life tends to be negative. Many people believe that they were born to suffer and subscribe to a life of negative behaviors that reflect their accepted misery. Sex for them becomes the only time that they are able to take a break from the emotional drama of their life. Sex calms the emotions. Why? Because the act of procreating is divine and the essential nature of man is a state of peace.

The limbic system was designed as a message system for the body. Sex calms, excites, creates happiness, induces joy, expands the sense of care, opens the energy centers of the body and increases the positive emotional energy between two people. Using sexual energy to balance the emotions is a technique that we will discuss in detail later in the text. Sex creates an emotional connection among people that facilitates a blending of the mental, physical and spiritual for activation of the memory of oneness. It is the holistic side of sex.

Chapter 3

Sexual Healing

To affect any type of healing in the body, the quantity and quality of energy flow must be changed. To achieve sexual healing, the mental, physical, emotional and spiritual energy must be balanced and channeled through the sexual organs and energy vortexes of the body. Activation of sexual healing energy will depend greatly on a person's sexual experiences. For example, there is a naturally low vibration or energy drain in cases of sexual abuse of any kind. The flow of energy may be even obsolete as a defense mechanism to these types of unhealed sexual wounds. Therefore, excessive amounts of sexual energy for a person suffering from sexual abuse will do more harm than good. For those suffering from sexual abuse, it is recommended to seek professional assistance with the mental, emotional, physical and spiritual imbalances to effectively internalize forgiveness.

On the opposite end of the spectrum is the excessive flow of sexual energy that is often driven by the egotistical animalistic nature of a person who has not found balance in the supply and demand of their sexuality. They often use sex as a cover up for other areas of perpetual unhappiness in their life. The hormonal releases in sexual orgasm can become addictive and leave many vital areas of life lacking the attention needed.

In a lifestyle guided by sexual healing, each sexual encounter is a source of empowerment for your highest good and the highest good of your partner. Sexual healing provides methods of reversing disease, regenerating the body, elevating the spiritual senses, balancing the emotions, increasing the mental faculties and manifesting positive components into the physical realm. Various techniques and states of awareness are a part of the sexual healing processes.

Sexual Reflexology
The sexual anatomy, the vagina and penis is just like the hands, feet, ears and scalp that have reflex points directly connected to nerve endings of the vital organs. In the wellness therapy of reflexology, providing focus and direct stimulation to reflex points on the body facilitates an increased flow of energy for the healing and regenerative processes. On the outer skin surface of the penis and the interior lining of the walls of the vagina, reflex points have been identified to be relative to the heart, lungs, spleen, pancreas, liver and kidneys.

The reflex points in both the vagina and the penis coincide with the heart and lungs in the upper region, the spleen, pancreas and liver in the middle region and the kidneys in the lower region. Therefore, in sexual healing the point of focus during intercourse is relative primarily to depth of penetration and positioning. When the penis penetrates deep within the vagina where it comes in contact with the cervix, it is energetically helping to regenerate the heart, lungs and the upper parts of the body in general. With a consciousness of sexual reflexology, both the male and the female facilitate this healing process for each other. When the depth of penetration lands mid-way the vagina, the female's spleen, pancreas and liver are nurtured. To stimulate energy of the male's liver, pancreas and spleen, the woman would concentrate the vaginal opening pull and caress around the midsection of the penis during her trust of motion. Stimulating the balancing properties of the kidneys is concentrated just inside the vaginal opening and at the base of the penis. However, the fact that sexual reflexology happens on a continuous basis during every sexual encounter is another reason why sex is an excellent physical health benefit.

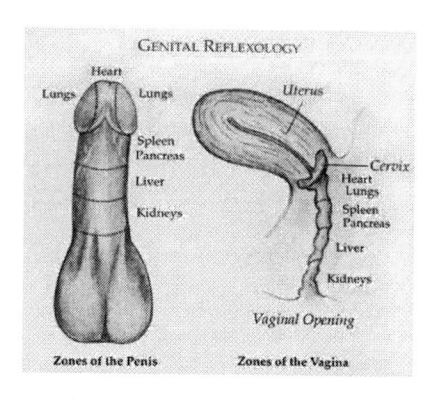

Genital Reflexology

Zones of the Penis: Heart, Lungs, Spleen/Pancreas, Liver, Kidneys

Zones of the Vagina: Uterus, Cervix, Heart/Lungs, Spleen/Pancreas, Liver, Kidneys, Vaginal Opening

Sexual reflexology extends farther beyond the noted organs in the diagram. Each region of the vagina and the penis also have holistic sexual functions in the form of key areas in the upper, middle, lower and full spans of the body. The upper region of the body in relationship to the divisions of the spinal column includes the head and neck. The middle area also known as the thoracic region includes the chest, the organs therein, the abdominal region and its organs. The lower region includes the pelvic area down to the feet. Therefore, if a couple will take up the use of sexual therapy using the conscious technique of depth of penetration, they are also able to assist in the health of their mate with focus on specific imbalances.

Examples of imbalances and symptoms of the organ systems in each of the four regions are listed in the following chart. If an ailment is physically manifesting in you or your mate, such as insomnia, the focus of penetration during sex would be deep within the vagina to stimulate the upper portions of the sexual anatomy. The same applies for the middle and lower points of focus as well.

UPPER	MIDDLE	LOWER	FULL BODY
• Headaches	• HBP	• Intestinal Issues	• Circulation
• Mental stress	• Respiratory Issues	• Reproductive organs	• Hormonal Imbalances
• Eye Issues	• Stomach	• Leg/Feet Issues	• Inflammation
• Insomnia	• Liver	• Pelvic Structure Regeneration	• Auto Immune Issues
	• Kidneys		• Detoxification

The use of sexual reflexology in holistic sexuality elevates the consciousness of the couple to a higher level of physical care for each other. Being able to provide sexual medicine to your divine reflection empowers the healer in you.

The use of sexual positioning in holistic sexuality adds an additional component of resources in this elevation of consciousness. There are numerous books and resources available for learning about sexual healing positions, if holistic sexuality is a lifestyle add-on that you and your mate will pursue, the investment would be very beneficial.

The sexual position is also a part of the point of concentration in the sexual healing process. For example, if your mate is having issues with the digestive system, choosing to nurture the energy of perfect health in the positions that best benefits the digestive organs will increase the capacity for the body to heal itself. These sexual positions are all about the motion and the physical therapy. When the body moves a certain way from an outside positive influence such as another body it facilitates internal massage that activates the mental and physical body of the particular organ. This increased specific motion provides a rhythmic toning and touch that all organs need for longevity. Sex is great. Even when people are not aware, just in the basic sexual positions, sex was designed to benefit the body in positive ways as you see in the positions below.

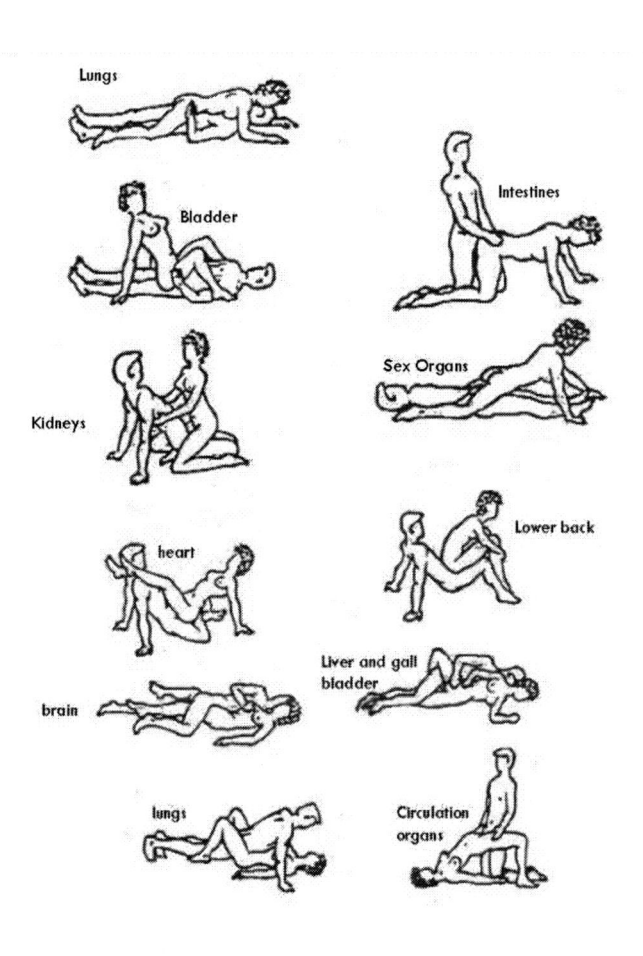

[Illustrations labeled: Lungs, Bladder, Intestines, Kidneys, Sex Organs, heart, Lower back, brain, Liver and gall bladder, lungs, Circulation organs]

Orgasm retention can be used by both male and female. It is a wellness technique that internally energizes and aligns the body with the preservation principles of holistic health. When something is preserved, it signifies that the owner recognizes the value and sacredness of the thing. An orgasm is a dissemination of energy throughout the body to enhance the continuation of the physical, mental, emotional and spiritual will to survive in the world for divine purpose.

Orgasm, as a glandular function ensures the continuation of the human species. If you have ever had an orgasm, and I hope that you have, you know that it feels like you are losing total control of your mind, body, senses, and everything about you. For a full five seconds, maybe a little longer orgasm allows the body to feel the full influx of universal energy running through your body and if you are honest with yourself, most will admit that they could not withstand the orgasmic state longer than a minute; you would lose your mind. The orgasm is a beautiful and intense state of energetic resonance that makes us want to keep experiencing this bliss over and over again.

Holistically, in order to not fall into the animalistic addiction of just having sex for the orgasmic feeling, it is necessary to internalize that without conscious consideration for the divine aspect of sex, one simply exists in a state of sexual dullness. This dullness will also be reflected in all other areas of life as well. It is all interconnected. However, to reduce and eliminate sexual dullness, the conscious use of orgasm retention aligns the entire mental, emotional and physical body with the beneficial energy patterns that are generated during sex.

Orgasm retention supplies the individual and the couple with many holistic health benefits. It restores energy to the body by creating a reserve that increases stamina and longevity. It increases mental clarity by quieting the mind and allowing for increased moments in the transcendental realm. During orgasm retention, your body speaks to you and communicates to you what the will needs to bring forth. That is why many people have great ideas and great conversation after sex. Orgasm retention eliminates premature ejaculations for men and women. When a woman uses orgasm retention, it helps her to maintain moisture levels in the vagina for a prolonged sexual experience. For men, orgasm retention also increases his longevity and this is beneficial especially when prolonged sex is required in certain aspects of sexual healing. Orgasm retention also works as a natural birthing rhythm method for couples who are not ready to procreate, by mastering this ejaculation control method during the regenerative phases of the menstrual cycle. Orgasm retention also increases spiritual sensuality by prolonging the state of mediumistic trance. We'll explain this type of trance momentarily. Being in a constant state of transcendence taps into the subconscious and unconscious realms of a person's will and this nurturing of the will aligns purpose with actions for successful manifestations.

To achieve orgasm retention during sex, allow the rhythmic motion of sex to build up to the point of feeling that the orgasm is about to happen and then calm the motion down by relaxing the body and mind with slow controlled breathing. When the potential orgasmic intensity slows and subsides, focus the energy in body to areas that are in need of balancing or begin visualization for mental, emotional or spiritual manifestations.

The most ignored aspect of human sexuality is its' ability to facilitate healing on all levels. Sexual union can be a transcendental experience that integrates two people into a state of wholeness.

Mediumistic Trance
Achieving sexual mediumistic trance is actually a natural occurrence during sex. Most people have experienced this level of trance. The ritual of sex often begins with the natural energy of attraction that exists between males and females. This energy activates the involuntary functions of the body in preparation for a sexual encounter. The body begins

to tense with anticipation of touch, the beginning acts of kissing and hugging release hormonal and glandular functions that increase penis blood flow, vaginal secretions and clitoral erection. Once the couple is engaged in the sexual act, there is a moment that is reached where everything that was in the full conscious awareness of the couple disappears. They no longer see the ceiling, they no longer hear noises in the room, they no longer smell the enchanting scent of the candles they lit to set the mood, and everything just halts for a few moments in time. If anything is heard, it is the breath or the sounds of their partner's moans, they only feel the motion of each other's body and everything else has literally left the building. This is the state of sexual mediumistic trance. Have you been there? It is a state of nonexistence where stuff starts fading out around you and the mind begins to leave the conscious realm and merges into sacred union with divine energy. The energy of the mind begin to delve into the subconscious and if one knows how to go deep enough, the unconscious can be accessed during this trance state as well.

To use mediumistic trance for the healing process involves visualization, affirmations and orgasm retention. If your mate is dealing with specific ailments in the body, mind, or spirit, this would be the time to envision them as whole and healthy.

Remember your thoughts affect the energetic outcome of those around you, and everyone is around you no matter the distance. If your partner is dealing with issues in their limbs where they have lost normal levels of mobility, you can visualize them running through a field of pansies or along a beautiful beach in a state of perfected health. If their heart and lungs are in need of regeneration from stress; these types of visualizations during this time of sex is very beneficial. What it does is impresses upon the mental faculty imprints of you and your partner by creating an energetic frequency of positive vibrations to the cellular realms of the physical body. You can liken it to redirecting the flow of water. Mediumistic trance can also be used to affect the physical presence of the family. For example, if the family is ready to move to a new home out of the city and there seem to be more obstacles than opportunities, sexual mediumistic trance can be used to envision this new home and the process of transition happening with ease and adequate resources. As a couple, you both begin to impregnate the subconscious and the unconscious mind with divine will. Divine will is in alignment with the family's purpose to move forward as a unit. This method of mental focus uses all of the aspects of healing available to man with the most power energy under human control and that is sexual energy.

Affirmations are an additional method of energy alignment confirmation that is used during mediumistic trance. What you say in your mind during sex is a direct reflection of your mental, spiritual and emotional health. Your thoughts have the ability to become the words that reveal your innermost self and your innermost self tells the world who you are. In holistic sexuality, that revelation points to the healer within. As you reach the semi-consciousness of mediumistic trance, brief affirmations can be mentally chanted with the same intentions as visualizations. You can speak words of health regeneration, positive movement in life, new thought pattern desires, help for loved ones, spiritual increase or anything that is needed to assist in your purpose living.

Sample affirmations:
- ☥ I see the god in you.
- ☥ We are in alignment with the energy of perfect health.
- ☥ I send healing light to your beautiful essence.
- ☥ I see the life we are destined to live.
- ☥ You are whole, happy and free.
- ☥ My body receives the light of your love.
- ☥ I seek reconnection to the divine.
- ☥ My spirit is joyful and grateful.
- ☥ I am seeking divine purpose.

☥   I am healed by your light energy.

Orgasm retention allows the couple to stay in mediumistic trance for longer periods of time. This is an additional benefit of orgasm retention. When a couple is able to sustain the presence of orgasmic energy, it helps to increase the potency of hormonal functions. In mediumistic trance, the greater the need, the longer the goal of mediumistic trance should be.

The mind and body is being released from mediumistic trance when full awareness of your surroundings become evident again. There is always a gradual decrease. Women naturally can maintain mediumistic trance longer because of the increased water levels in female tissues that generates a higher level of electricity. So, if she tends to remain in that euphoric state longer than the man, he is encouraged to continue to lovingly support her trance state with silent encouragement.

Sexual Healing Tempo and Tones
Both partners are able to enjoy a prolonged state of trance with the use of voice inflections, vibration pitches and specific sounds to enhance the body's reaction during sex. Think about the musical note scale.

The reason music is a joy during sex is because the vibration of the tones facilitate a form of energetic instructions for various parts of the body. These vibrations depending on the pitch will affect certain organs, hormones, nerves and physical areas of the body. High pitched tones affect the upper part of the body, all areas of the shoulders, neck and head.. In sex when the music or the voiced sounds of your partner is high, it causes a release of hormonal secretions that intensify the sexual desire and a concentrated intention of pleasing your partner. The music that provides these tones best is jazz and meditation music. High tones will concentrate the sexual energy in the upper part of the body therefore providing the platform for longevity in the mediumistic trance state.

Mid ranged tones affect the mid section of the body where the vital organs are housed in the abdomen and the back. The gentle massage of the internal organs during sex and a consistent pitch of mid toned sounds have a regenerative aspect in the healing process. These mid tones relax, soothe, filter and tone the cellular structure of the liver, kidneys, lungs, intestines, stomach, spleen and heart.

The music that provides these tones best is R & B, nature sounds and the blues. The mid tones also prolong mediumistic trance because of the relaxation mode of the vibration in the soothing sound of your mate's voice or music that radiates the mid section.

The low tones will stimulate the reproductive system and enhance its maximum potential; however, it will also increase the intensity for the physical body to achieve orgasm. Low tones that center around what we call bass tones as in slow tempo rap music without the lyrics, love songs like The Isley Brothers and bass toned cultural drum music directly affect the penis, uterus, vagina, ovaries and testicles. To increase productivity in the reproductive system, this music can also be listened to when a couple has the intention to conceive.

Living a holistic sexuality lifestyle is a learning process. To be able to heal yourself and your mate(s) involves a practice of the principles of holistic sexuality and the application of the methods of interrelating that bring the balance of harmony through trust and open communication. Holistic Sexuality is another one of our built in medicine makers supplied by the creator to give us a full life that speaks to immortality.

Chapter 4

Mental and Emotional Maintenance Through Relationship Intelligence

Holistic sexual energy is designed to direct the mind to higher levels of consciousness by assisting seekers in finding balance, creating an unconditional bond and a spiritual devotion in relationships.

Holistic sexuality involves more than just you and a partner. Holistic Sexuality involves you and your relationship with the universe. If you cannot diligently ingest universal oneness in all that you see, feel, hear, taste, and know you will have a difficult time applying yourself to the holistic way of anything. Developing a metaphysical and quantum view of every relationship that you exist in is key for wholeness on every level. There are three primary relationship masteries that enrich your level of purification from a dysfunctional relationship lifestyle: honesty, Relationship Intelligence, and consistency in the flow of change. The foundation for changing your sexual lifestyle is complete, open, and honest communication with your mate(s). Society has taught us to live in a constant state of fear. People who are afraid of the consequences of their actions will tell lies. Liars approach sex with the wrong intentions. Liars don't want to be responsible for the powerful energetic exchange that truth and honesty brings. Liars want to maintain a comfortable flow of energy by not dealing with how they really feel and their preferences in life and relationships. People who are afraid of rejection and who live with insecurities will put forth their best face and pretend to be, want and do things that are not in alignment with their greatest good or the greater good of their mate(s).

Dishonesty in a sexual relationship creates mental and emotional dysfunctional states of being. It causes a stress that lingers in the thoughts. This lingering produces a mental pressure that makes it hard to trust and not being able to trust your mate(s) leaves mental scars that require a lot of work to heal even if you move forward out of the relationship. Without a purification process from mate to mate that involves forgiveness and rebuilding trust, a person will find themselves in new relationships repeating the same dysfunctional behavior that drove them from the last relationship. It is an aspect of the laws of attraction, where you attract to you what is in the inner most depths of your subconscious self, even if your surface self appears to be ok. The wounds don't heal on their own, the individual or the couple must take time to establish and complete a healing process. Depending on the mental and emotional maturity of the individuals, this could take months, years, decades or a lifetime. Dishonesty also breeds low energy levels in the relationship and these will cause mental fatigue which often results in the animalistic nature of sex becoming the norm between the couple. They go through the motions of sex. For one, it's for the physical pleasure and for the other, sex becomes an obligation without pleasure. Some people operate in this state for a lifetime. The mental strain of dishonesty makes a person think negatively about themselves and negatively of other people. Thoughts are also energy exchanges. You are what you think you are and you are what you think others are and vice versa. You can become on an energetic and subconscious level what someone constantly thinks about you and communicates to you. So the healing and maintenance of a healthy mentality in a sexual relationship is only achieved through open and honest communications.

Honesty in a sexual relationship has the power to preserve the divine intentions of the couple when they come together. They are able to talk about their sexual preferences. They have no fear in expressing to their mates the type of family structure they want. This type of honesty creates a high vibration of energy in the relationship and offers security. The mental and emotional balance that couples produce can be shared with others as an example of good relationship intelligence. This interrelating removes the fear. It establishes a permanent trust factor and brings forth that which is spiritually correct.

Relationship Intelligence

Our entire existence is our relationships with the universe around us. We would hope that these relationships have the intention of working towards our greater good. That is why is it good to stop sometimes to evaluate and reevaluate our personal relationships with the people, places and material things that make up the majority of our everyday life.

Relationship Intelligence is necessary in order for many to move forward in their spiritual elevation. This is one of the most vital areas to have in balance for a holistic lifestyle. If everyone around you is dysfunctional and you are in constant contact with them, spiritual ascension and peace will be almost impossible.

Wholeness means having balance in your mental, physical, emotional and spiritual self that no one can shake. The only reason we form relationships is to join with others who will add substance to the fulfillment of our divine purpose. With this in mind, they must add to all of your holistic aspects of life.

Some questions to ask yourself in relation to the people in your life:
- ☥ What does this person add to my mental progress?

- ☥ Does this person add to my emotional balance?
- ☥ Do I receive spiritual nourishment and peace from their presence in my life?
- ☥ How does this relationship enhance me physically?
- ☥ Is this relationship a contribution to my overall greater good?

I think you know what to do with your answers. Remember your divine self knows what is best for self.

A very vital relationship that you must find balance in when your consciousness is awakened is the relationship with SELF.

There's a new fact about personal relationships that I want to share: you can only give to someone else what you have. What I mean by this is if you are dysfunctional, emotional and always have problems perplexing you, then that is what you have to give. If you are spiritually attuned, living a balanced life, physically healthy and mentally progressive, then that is what you have to give. Self cannot deceive self, the truth will always come to face attempted deception as frustration.

Taking an honest look at yourself, ask, "What do I have to give in my relationships with others? What values do I bring to the relationships in my life?"

Self Relationship Check: Let's see what you're working with!
- Are you connected to your spiritual source?
- Do you listen to your first mind?
- Do you spend time in deep contemplation/meditation?
- Are you an independent thinker?
- Are you physically healthy?
- Do you like your body?
- Do you enjoy sex?
- Are you financially stable?
- Are you able to observe your emotional responses without attachment?
- Are you able to maintain an emotional equilibrium when you are upset?
- Do you have a healthy thought pattern about sex?
- Can you respect and accept others even when what they want is not what you want?

Another new fact to consider in relationships is that you attract that which you are. After surveying your answers to the above questions, apply them to some of the people that you have close relationships with and you will find some similarities in the answers.

If you get too many no answers this might be a time of reevaluation and restructuring of self. Get yourself together first, that way, what you have to give is the best of you. And contrary to popular belief, relationships do not have to be dysfunctional and full of drama. There is a life of peace available to the wise that are ready to KNOW their divine SELF.

Living in harmony with our divine reflection in the form of the masculine divine or feminine divine energy is a special rites of passage. In the early stages of relationship intelligence, people find themselves in an immature in mental, emotional and spiritual state of development. Move to a higher understanding of male/female personal relationships through the knowledge of mastering the levels of energy manifestations that people possess. There are several types of personalities that your mate could possess that will make them either appeal to you or repel you based on the level of awareness you are at in your spiritual development. These energy manifestations can be seen in both females and males.

The Nurturer cares on all levels and provides the soft essence of motherly love. They may or may not have much to give on the material level, however, they surrender their life line to ensure others are well cared for.

The Planner knows how to organize everything and is the master motivator. They want you to do your best and will assist in organizing with you for your purpose work. They provide a great example of what having it together means.

The Divine One not only bedazzles the physical eye, they also stimulate the very spiritual core of those they come in contact with. They walk with a light that says you are special and I honor you as my divine reflection.

The Ruler knows how to run the show and can take care of everything and everybody. Their words rule through the manifestations of their actions.

The Friend is the one who listens and supports unconditionally above all else. They stand by your side and offer what they have to assist where needed.

The Talker communicates on all levels in the relationship. They are involved; and fully participate in the relationship on a verbal level.

The Thinker is the logical one who seeks the lesson in all they do. They are constantly intrigued by and involved in mental expansion. Their scholarly ways are founded in the need to know for the greater experience of life.

The Seer uses their sense of visualization and seeing is doing as their platform for receiving life in all its many facets. They find pleasure in knowing through sight.

The Doer is the hands on person who loves to get up and go. They are the ones who like to keep their lives moving. The Doer learns and thrives by their hands, feet and being mobile.

The Song is a rhythmic person who lives in the flow of the melodies of life. They love being surrounded by music and it is their greatest form of relaxation, motivation and dedication.

Interpersonal people are outgoing and enjoy the crowd. They will take moments of silence and one on one time but their preference is the group.

Intrapersonal people are the quiet type who likes being alone. They enjoy the one on one relationship and are content with not doing much outside of the necessities in life. They like what they like and prefer to do things their own way.

Do you see a part of yourself in any of these energy essences? Actually, the person who is balanced mentally, emotionally, spiritually and physically will see themselves in a few of these. They will also be able to share the light that they are with their divine reflection because they will attract who they are!

Male/Female Relationships
A male and female relationship that reflects harmony, trust, security, support, purpose and growth is the most sacred of unions. Choosing to become a couple is a natural connection between man and woman. To create this bond of longevity ties directly into preservation of culture, the creation of social normality, the potential to increase economic sufficiency, and the continuation of proliferation as a standard of life. These great benefits also come with responsibilities, roles and goals to share.

In my many years of marriage, I have found that there are 12 Key Formulas to a successful relationship, that if addressed fully with the best of intentions and honesty, couples are able to flow in their lives together with the support that nurtures their individual selves and their lives as a divine unit. In an effort to build and fortify the ever changing bond that reconnects the spirit of two individuals who are seeking spiritual harmony, the internalization and complete implementation of these relationship principles and practices will make the commitment a rewarding relationship for the rest of your life and your love for each other will be remembered for generations to come.

Formula 1
Life Purpose

Before you consider marriage or a committed relationship with another person, it is critical that you work on your whole self as the primary relationship in your life.

Consider what you saw and learned from the adult relationships in your childhood. How did this shape you? Consider the things that you know are dysfunctional about yourself and how you have functioned in relationships in the past. Put yourself to the test with a few important questions.

What are my reasons for wanting a personal relationship at this time in my life? Make a list of ten or more reasons.

What are the things I want to get a chance to do in this life that will support my hopes and wishes? Make a list of 10 or more and label the top 5.

All your answers must sit well with your spirit, if your intuition gives you a doubt about your intention, you need to meditate on what is really coming through to you about this aspect of yourself.

If you are currently in a relationship and contemplating marriage, you will want to have your mate to make a list for themselves also. You will then need to sit down together in complete honesty and share your lists with each other. Talk about the different reasons for wanting marriage and how these reasons compliment and differ from each other. Take the time to share all the things that you want to do and be in this life time. Then choose the three that you must do before you leave this physical realm.

Next is one of the most important parts of your beginnings together as possible life mates. After sharing the top three aspirations on your lists, the question to ask each other is can you and will you say "yes" to all of these aspirations and offer 110% support to them when the time comes for your partner to fulfill that part of their purpose.

Learning and being able to say yes is one of the most important duties you will have in a personal relationship. Saying yes to offer your support in helping anyone fulfill that which sets well with their spirit is divine encouragement for them to be in alignment with who they are in the universe. However, remember that being in alignment with yourself first helps to bring balance to life.

Formula 2
Love: The Energy of Connection

Love is a vibration of the creator that is within everything that exists in this universe. It is an energy that is neither created nor destroyed. I was taught by a power-full healer that love is a given. In relationship to the energy of love and the people in our lives, if one has opened themselves to the unifying oneness of the creator, to love someone is a non-issue. Being in alignment with the energy of love, you know through your wisdom that it is critical to meet people where they are and send positive vibrations to the things that they do to fulfill their purpose. If they are on their path; then balance will prevail and it will be all good. Developing a real concept of love is not just dwelling in the emotional baggage of the words, "I love you"; it requires a new thought process and understanding.

Love is the energy that allows you to move your arms, feel the warmth of the sun and it is the energy that governs your understanding that life is sacred and requires care. Love is the reason you are able to look into someone else's eyes and recognize they are a valuable human with purpose. Love is the energy that makes you aware of the moon and stars. Love is the energy that connects you to the beauty of the trees, flowers and waters of the Earth.

Love, as energy, provides an existence of the unconditional. You have no control over love in its truest form, in fact, you are the energy of love in its truest form. This concept will be difficult for many to grasp or even accept, however, for those wise ones among us who dwell in the cellular memory of the perfection of the divine, this concept of truth will set well with the peace that your soul is.

These inspirations in love can also assist you in moving beyond the dysfunctional hypocrisies that people often find themselves in surrounding the misconception of love. "I love you", but there is abuse, mistrust, fear, greed, unhappiness, doubt etc…

Practice feeling the vibration of love (the energy) in association with everything about yourself.

You don't need validation from anyone; your degree of self love should be immeasurable.

Don't be arrogant; fulfill your desire to share the positivity that you feel about yourself with all that you meet.

Be pleasant to be around.

Take time for relaxation and pampering at least twice a month.

Spend time everyday in meditation.

Look up at the sun and deliberately breathe in the air and allow the warm energy to saturate your skin.

Live the Principles of MAAT:
Truth - Speak it each time you open your mouth so that those who hear your words learn divine alignment.

Reciprocity - Giving all that you want in return is an example of the unconditional.

Propriety - Be a physical, mental, emotional and spiritual example of what you want to see in your community.

Order - Innerstand your responsibility as a protector of Nature, live life in accordance with the time given to all creation to complete its cycle.

Balance - There is no me without you, there is no us without nature, develop a consciousness to meet all where they are without judgments or expectations that are not in alignment with divine law.

Righteousness- Have the courage, condition the body and mind to have the strength to do right, live right and learn the qualities required for divine defense and awesome offense when it is needed in the community.

Harmony - This is love manifested unconditionally, this is a peace that is unshakable, this is what you will find when MAAT is present in the everyday existence of who you are.

Stop sometimes to write down your thoughts on things that are happening in your life and evaluate where you need balance or where you need to spend more time working on a certain area.

Love never dies; it is an energy that has always existed to connect the protectors of nature to the creator.

Formula 3
Commitment

Commitment in a relationship is taking on the emotional, physical, mental and spiritual responsibility for yourself and others. Commitment has to be shown in what you do, not what you say.

Once a clear pattern of love for yourself has been established and you are living it daily, consciously practicing and sharing it unconditionally with all that cross your path, then you are most likely ready to think about possible commitment to align yourself with someone else.

Commitment is being able to be flexible for the changes in life. It is honoring the ever changing cycles of life that present themselves as progress.

Formula 4
The Physical Bodies

It is important to maintain physical and emotional balance in the relationship. Each person has to internalize the following and consider this when the energy of possession and jealousy rears its head at times on the relationship.

You cannot possess me for I belong to myself, but while we both wish it, I give you that which is mine to give.

You cannot command me, for I am a free person, but I shall serve you in those ways you require and the honeycomb will taste sweeter coming from my hand.
- *Sankrit saying*

With this in mind, you will want to put emphasis on caring for your body. Consider how your ideal body looks to you. Are you there? If so, a part of your holistic health regiment should be to maintain your healthy body, however, be fully aware that physical changes are going to take place as you age and those changes are a part positive maturity. If not, then part of the work you do on yourself should be developing a lifestyle that will help you achieve your beautiful body. Another vital aspect of the physical body in a holistic relationship is maintaining a healthy sexuality, and being satisfied with your physical will assure positive sensuality.

Formula 5
Developing the Spirit

It would be ideal for people to have all their stuff together before entering into a personal relationship. However, in most cases the beginning of a relationship is riding on emotions, money or sexual attraction in western society. None of these make for a holistic relationship with longevity. The best foundation for any relationship, especially one that you are looking to establish for longevity, is to maintain a connection to your spiritual source. Knowing that you and your mate are divine energy, that same energy that permeates the universe and causes the sun to do its work, the vegetables to grow in your garden, the ocean to maintain its balance in the world is the same energy that allows your heart to beat each moment. You and your mate are the source of life connected to all. If you are able to see at every moment the divine in your mate, you will find your relationship growing and fulfilling. For example, if you know your mate to be a divine being meaning you see the god in them, and express your gratitude in every encounter you have with them, it creates a peace in your life that enriches your commitment.

Another way of staying spiritually connected is to spend time quiet and alone. There must always be some time that you take to yourself to reflect on life and where you are in it at the moment. Both you and your mate should take some time each year to just go away for a few days from all that is familiar to just be and do what you want or need to do. I think the popular term for it now is me time. Remember this is not a time for frivolous endeavors but a time of spiritual enrichment.

Develop a relationship with your inner wisdom, intuition and discipline for consistency. Trust in everything that your first mind tells you. It will never steer you wrong. It is the inner wisdom talking to you and waiting with great anticipation for you to embrace what is for you. Stop going back and forth with your thoughts and just listen. However, if by chance you do get confused and can't remember what your first mind said, then take it to your mate and let their first mind help you decide. This way you will also find balance in being part of the greater whole and oneness of the creator.

Formula 6
Communication

Communication must always be open, honest and constant. Communication is the indication of the need we have for each other. What kind of communicator are you? Do you communicate more effectively with body language, letter writing, straight talk, and/or facial expressions? Learn to define your way of communicating and that of your mate's so there are no misunderstandings in your inner and outer relations to each other.

There will be times when your relationship will need effective communication in an emotional state. First off, if you are in a negative emotional state, it is best to keep quiet as communication at such a time will be driven by erratic thoughts. Unclear thinking can lead to all kinds of things coming out your mouth, so just be quiet until you are able to think clearly about what you want to communicate in a way that is in alignment with your spiritual self.

Open communication can be difficult because most people have learned to shut down when communication or personal thoughts become difficult to express through perceived expectations in a relationship. Open communication means having the courage to express what is in the mind as it relates to harmony, sharing, problem solving, understanding, truth and progress.

Harmony Communication are those conversations you have about building and maintaining life together. This is your merging of goals, desires and fulfilling dreams.

Sharing Communication is talking to each other about your experiences in life. What you learned in the world for the day, what encounters made an impression on you and how you felt about it. Sharing Communication provides an outlet to solidify your lessons in life and express how these learning moments influenced or changed you.

Problem Solving Communication is an exercise in accessing your higher self. When a challenge presents itself in the relationship, to have the courage to speak on it without an emotional upheaval is operating on a higher level of consciousness than the average person. Problem Solving Communication must first begin with personal reflection and gratitude. If you have a situation that occurs in your relationship that causes you stress and frustration, the first question to ask yourself is why? Why does this bother me? Is it because of my emotional immaturity? Does this problem cause a physical threat or harm to the family? Once you are able to pinpoint why the situation bothers you, then you are ready to go within and bring forth a solution based on your inner wisdom. After you and the god in you have talked about the problem and you now have some solutions to bring to the table, then you are ready to talk with your mate and intelligently communicate for progress. Anytime something in your relationship appears to be a problem, accept ownership of it; because when something bothers you, it is a personal problem.

Understanding Communication is having the ability to listen and appreciate commonalities and differences. Each person, as an individual, will always have different thoughts and ideas about life and the many ways to live it according to their own purpose. Respect for these differences when they arise is what understanding is about. This is your vow of commitment to support your mate in the things that set well with their spirit, and remember the spirit of a person is what moves them through life with purpose.

Truth Communication is courage. The courage to bring forth your emotional, mental, spiritual and physical alignments at every moment in your relationship is only facilitated through the minds of the transcendent souls among us. This is often the most difficult in every relationship. This communication is only achieved through the elimination of all fear in life. I encourage you to go through the uncomfortable feelings when you have to communicate something that you think will not set well with your mate and stand with the knowledge that it is ok to be who you are. Your truth belongs to you and is never based on what someone else dictates. Be who the Creator created you to be and use your divine words to build, encourage, change and stand strong. Truth Communication also has a gentler side. It is also ok to speak your truth in teaching those lessons in life that have made you stronger and more vibrant, people are encouraged by other people. If your mind leads you to share in this manner, don't hesitate someone is waiting to receive.

Progress Communication is being able to talk with your mate about everything, because remember, you both are striving to grow together and that includes being able to listen and receive without judgment or criticism. There is a forth coming section on Constant Planning, and progress communication is that time you spend together talking about your achievements and planning for your future.

Communication is a growth process for every couple especially in western culture. Stay encouraged as you learn effective communication.

Formula 7
Constant Planning

As a family you should find yourselves in constant communication with each other on your thoughts, feelings, physical bodies, aspirations and your daily lives. As the universe is in constant motion, so are we as divine energy. We have the gift of intelligence to use for divine purpose here on earth. With this in mind, as a family, you should be constantly planning to do what is being put before you as a part of your purpose and responsibility. You should schedule family meetings and keep records of what the goals and aspirations are for each member of the family. Then work and support each other in achieving those goals. Never remain complacent. The creator is in constant motion as an example for us. Constant planning for most families will include adding children to the family.

Formula 8
Children are the rewards of life.

Children are one of the primary reasons why strong and stable relationships are vital to our communities. The number of children the family produces is in divine alignment with the creator's will. Sometimes we have something to say about it and sometimes not. However, the reality is that most families do not have ten plus children like our early ancestors did. The rearing of the children should be talked about prior to the children coming into the physical world. It would be ideal for mother to be able to stay home and breast feed the children until their little systems are ready to travel on their own, but if that is not possible for your family, then systems of care where the work is equally distributed needs to be worked out.

The holistic education of the children in the ways of the ancestors, cultural norms, healthy eating practices, and the use of information received in an outside school setting are all things to consider when planning and raising children. When you are faced with the issue of discipline and correcting the behavior of your child, remember that until the age of eight children operate on pure emotion. So be patient with them and give them the innerstanding of only being in this physical realm for the few short years, they don't know a whole lot. Provide for them the example of how to live and know that they are their own people and they will never be just like you so encourage them to embrace their uniqueness.

Formula 9
Family Financial Health

Along with children and possibly before, many families today focus a lot of their attention on finances. The buzz is that this is the reason for most single parent homes and divorces in the western societies. King Kwabena F. Ashanti says, *"Families must pool their monies together for economic developments and assistance to each other."*

Before marriage and all during, the following should be addressed for the longevity and prosperity of the family. Rate your financial situation in life on a scale of 1 – 10 then write 3 things that could make your financial situation better. Take time to evaluate what the family income is being used for. If the family is in more need of income to progress the family, know that two incomes are better and multiple streams of income are best. Every person is endowed with a gift of talent, and it is always good to make money doing what you love to do. So think about those things that you are good at and make a stream of income for the family. Everyone should have a stream of income including the children and although they do not work outside of the home, they can work for the family in helping to grow and sell food, answer sales calls, run errands, etc.

Financial education is a requirement for all in the family, the more you know finances and economics, the better you can do with money management, sensible spending habits, obtaining financial security, creating cash flow businesses, eliminating debt, making investments in real estate and business, savings for emergencies and the children, multiple streams of income and being an entrepreneur.

Financial meetings need to be held in the family at least every three months so that everyone can remain on the same page with the financial health of the family. Avoid emotional spending, this is where you spend money to try and dissipate negative vibrations or emotional imbalance. For times like this, communicate and get to the source of the issue to heal instead of putting bandages on problems.

The thoughts you put into the financial health of the family is what the family will receive in return. So keep your thoughts positive and in alignment with prosperity.

Formula 10
A Healthy Lifestyle

If you have any of the common addictive vices that add stress to the family's health, then it would be wise to take the steps necessary for personal change. Eliminate drugs, alcohol, smoking, household chemicals, clutter and uncleanness. Eat organic when and where you can. Again, educate yourself on as many avenues of holistic health so that you are able to heal your family in a time of need.

Formula 11
Spiritual Sexuality

Sexual Spirituality is a component that should be with you throughout the course of your lives together. The sacredness of this energy exchange should be used to procreate and strengthen each other physically, mentally, emotionally and spiritually. You should develop rituals that are meaningful to you and express your desire to share sacred sexual time. Positive affirmations can be developed to express to your mate and the creator of what your intentions are each time you join together. It is important that you communicate before and after sex to become more in tune with your mates' preferences. Be adventurous and stable at the same time if a certain aspect of the union works, use it often, however, don't be afraid to follow your divine intuition when spirit leads you to try something new. Sex is a beautiful energy exchange and it will be beneficial if future generations are taught correctly of its sacredness and the gift of the responsibility to procreate for the survival of nature.

Formula 12
The Tough Questions

Every marriage has moments of strain and challenge, but that is just what it should be, a moment, if the two are in alignment with themselves and nature. However, there are a few situations in marriage that are not unique to you, because everything that is already was, and this might just happen to be your turn to go through it. We present these just as questions that really need to be addressed before marriage, only you and your mate can answer them.

How do I feel about my spouse having intimate relationships with others?

Am I open to polygamy or polyandry?

What will I do if the family is ever in a financial crisis?

How will I deal with the death of my mate or child?

How much involvement will I allow our families to have in the marriage?

How will I deal with my mate's social life outside of the home?

What do I do if I decide I want to leave the marriage?

Sincerely incorporating the 12 Formulas of a Holistic Relationship throughout your union will help you to use your wisdom to constantly stay aligned with your root purpose.

Last in the maintaining mental and emotional balance in relationship intelligence is to perfect the flow of change with consistency. The nature of the creator is change and as a part of creation men and women also change on a daily basis. Life is supposed to be fluid and free flowing, and by design we are mobile beings with high intelligence. When something around us changes, we have the capacity to learn from it, live with it and nurture the newness that comes into being. Having this frame of mind about male and female relationships reveals a level of character development that is above the norm.

One should expect change in their mates, it is a sign of growth on some level, though you may not necessarily understand when change happens, it is still ok to allow the process to unfold without surrounding it with negative energy and comparisons of how it doesn't fit into what you think what your mate ought to be doing.

How do you handle change that causes an emotional response of discomfort?

Trust.

Trust that because you and your mate have been working on yourselves and you have made solid commitments to the relationship that you are able to openly communicate about any new directions in life. Mastering the trust factor relieves the frustration of wanting to control something that you have no control over. Trusting your mate says to them, you are a divine being who is fully capable of directing your own life as we share this path together. And even if our paths take on different directions, we leave each other in peace embracing and internalizing with gratitude all of the life lessons we have grown with together. Trust allows you to let go of worry, frustration and fear. Trust encourages you to refer back to the 12 Formulas of nurturing a relationship just in case there is emotional regression.

Be open to change for yourself and change with your mate. This is a vital support component in every relationship. Most people follow their heart in the things they choose to do in life and listening to that inner voice is a treasure waiting to be revealed.

Incorporating Relationship Intelligence takes time and effort. If you have attracted who you are, then you now have a good idea of how much time it will take to develop into who you and your mate are according to your purposes.

Chapter 5

Establishing the Divine Family Structure

Divine Family Structures

Man and woman together create the balance of procreation in the universe. One cannot and should not exist without the other. The divine structure of these relationships is where most people have complications and develop emotional problems. Most people have a problem with being honest about what they really want in their relationships to be able to live in harmony with their procreator(s).

Ask yourself, what is the best family structure for me to be able to fulfill my divine purpose in this life time?

Monogamy?
Polygamy?
Polyandry?
Polyamory?

A spiritually correct union is free flowing and committed. It is time to stop being dishonest in relationships. It is perfectly fine to be in a monogamous relationship. It is perfectly fine to be in a polygamous relationship. It is perfectly fine to be in a polyandry relationship. It is perfectly fine to be in a polyamory relationship. All of these relationships work if people come together with the best of intentions. It is time to be clear about what is best for you in your personal relationships.

Relationships can only radiate freely if they are centered in the unconscious awareness known as trust. The balance of trust in a relationship is honesty, and honesty is relating to each other as things really are and not how you want them to be. To be honest, it takes courage because although honesty is talked about and expected in relationships, this society has made dishonesty the norm. To facilitate courage in a relationship, one must have the strength to choose your true self over what others want you to be. Most people do not have the courage to vibrate in this capacity when it comes to their relationships. They are afraid to take on the responsibility of the high vibration that honesty brings. This fear is breeding the continuation of lies, deceit, cheating, sneaking and breaking up over something as trivial as five minutes of sex. This is a hindrance when it comes to manifesting divine potential. It serves no purpose to be dishonest; it only disrupts relationships and causes unnecessary pain and suffering. (Sherwood 1992) To be honest and courageous is to say yes to the balance of life and this affirms your ability to radiate freely in any relationship that you choose.

Let us take a moment to look at family structures from a spiritual and holistic point of view. There are four main family structures to choose from and because of religion and man's idiosyncrasies, we have not been "allowed" or taught to openly explore these viable spiritual unions. The four family structures are monogamy, polygamy, polyandry and polyamory. Now the first thing I want you to know is that if an individual is not living life with a mastery of truth, propriety, order, balance, righteousness, reciprocity, harmony and has not established an unshakable foundation of self love, none of the family structures will work effectively for an extended period of time.

MONOGAMY is having a commitment and sexual relationship with one partner. Once you have yourself together, you attract and choose a mate that will be the sole partner to assist and support you in fulfilling your divine purpose and to share your gifts to assist them to fulfill their divine purpose on the life journey. Any situation that causes you not to see the divine in them and the divine in yourself is immediately worked through with the intention of moving forward together.

In doing research on true monogamous couples, it was very difficult to find a couple who had been faithful to the practice and guidelines of monogamy for the full extent of their relationship. However, in several surveys, once couples realized that their commitment, time and energy are best spent nurturing each other is when the courage and discipline that is needed in a monogamous relationship became a true lifestyle.

A misconception of monogamy also lies in the happily ever after myth that is instilled in the minds of modern societies that are set up on religious dogma and fairytales. Yes it is possible to find your one true love, however, the natural sexual instincts that humans possess which validates the natural attraction between man and woman makes monogamy the one family structure that requires a great amount of discipline. All extramarital relationships that cause problems for couples are centered mainly on sex. Even sexual confusion takes place in monogamous relationships when the sex drive of one partner changes and the other partner develops sexual frustration because of the restrictions of monogamy.

Monogamy is also a form of protection and a good stabilizer in relationships. Protection in the sense that an unconditional commitment and bond between a man and woman to offer their total support of each other's purpose for an extended period of time forms a stable environment for growth and self centered nourishment.

Monogamy as the basic format of relationships in human nature is a great start for any couple, because once two people have mastered the care, support and commitment for one other person, they may find themselves then willing to share this profound knowledge and lifestyle with others by teaching others the benefits of monogamy and how to live it well.

POLYGAMY in its intended form of truth is when the divine masculine in his God Essence has acquired the knowledge of a spiritual discipline system that equips him with the mental, physical, emotional and spiritual strategies to provide more than one woman with the essence of his divinity that will assist each one on their journey to fulfilling their purpose. The women who are best fitted for this type of family structure are those who have become in tune with their divine feminine faculty and are able to see, feel and know their sister wives as divine reflections of themselves. They live by the truth that there is no me without you. Polygamy is recorded in time among all people, cultures and societies. Among a few of the religious and cultural organizations in the world, this system is still a viable part of communities today.

Polygamy as a family structure as observed among local, national and international groups is a cooperative of support and potential growth. Because women make up the majority of the family structure, the balancing of the feminine divine requires a great deal of time and effort from the male energy. Therefore, men who choose this family structure should be strong in the spiritual will first. This gives them the ability to build a family of women who reflect the spiritual character that is necessary to promote emotional maturity, positive mental enrichments and unconditional physical care for each member of the family.

POLYANDRY is based on the spiritual elevation of the divine feminine who has reached a vibration level of a true Goddess. She attracts and selects her divine masculine reflections and because she is the master nurturer, the sensual essence of feminine energy, a visionary for community change and an organizer out of this world, she is able to bring together men who will work together and support each other without fear or jealousy because they KNOW that she has a limitless source of energy that will work with them in fulfilling their divine purpose as men.

Why polyandry? To speak to the truth of oneness. To develop a holistic system of life that includes giving acceptance to divine reconnections of the creator's manifestations in physical form which assist in developing a network of healing workers with a common goal to ensure the survival of balance throughout eternity. As the goddess bestowed upon those made in her image to be the ones to nurture and continue life in the physical realm, it is she who has been given the responsibility to carry forth the reunification of the One.

Polyandry as a family structure requires that all parties love, think, breathe, know and live the principle of universal oneness. It is vital to set aside patriarchal western conditioning about relationships and embrace the matriarchal concept of existence.

These are some proven steps to a successful Polyandry Family Structure.

When considering polyandry as a family structure it is vital to reveal your current family make up.

The family must have a strong spiritual and cultural lifestyle with a firm system of spiritual guidance and dedication to living the knowledge of oneness.

The family must be seekers of balance in all that they do and they will best achieve this by effective communication and a cycle of quality time which includes family meetings and supporting each other's endeavors. It is vital to constantly speak words of understanding and patience.

The family must have an open line of communication to express their emotions to one another without the personal attachments that hinder growth.

There is an emphasis on healthy living and longevity. The family lives with a consistent regimen of exercise and cleanliness. Taking care of the body and teaching the children all that they should know to maintain excellent health.

Intimacy is a given, it is a sacred ritual of bonding and procreating. It is the unifying force that connects, enriches, and allows for the tasting of blissfulness of the divine essence. Enjoy and know that everything happens in divine time. Procreation is desired by the creator and will be a family decision.

For women who are considering this family structure, focus on your goals and being in alignment with all those things that enhance your life. Here are a few questions to begin the process of knowing if polyandry is right for you.

What are three things that you want to do in life above all else?

What are your strengths, weaknesses, and skills?

What do you have to offer multiple mates that would render you acceptable for this divine system of companionship?

Why do you choose polyandry?

Setting family goals is also important in polyandry. Good family goals where a polyandry family structure would be beneficial include maintaining financial independence, achieving sovereignty, food production, nation building and spiritual development.

There are also various types of living arrangements that can be considered for the family. Give your prospective spouses a choice in living locations. Either the family can live in one established home or each spouse can provide a home in a different location that may be relevant to his work, career or living preference.

With the knowledge that the children are the rewards of life and they are the future that we build the holistic foundation for, the family should strive to do only those things that will benefit the infinite generations to come. In polyandry, the concept is, your children are our children and we all work together to secure and train them to embrace the god/goddess within themselves to continue the will of the creator which is experiencing and fulfilling divine purpose.

When man and woman join together in a spiritual bond and the cultivation of procreation is the result, it is a rite of passage. In the realm of living as a spiritual entity the immediate cultivation of the spiritual, physical, emotional and mental development of the child begins with mother, father and the entire family upholding the principles of divine law.

Truth will be crucial in the development of the child, know the truth to be taught at every stage of development.

Reciprocity is achieved with a mind of giving unconditionally, put all of your positive energies into everything that is spoken, made and intended for the child. This is done knowing that what is put into the energy of the child will manifest back to the family and the world.

Propriety is when the parents take on the role of procreators it is important for the community to see and know that the development of all aspects of the child is taking place.

Order is exercising patience in the development and training of the child and providing the opportunities for the appropriate rites of passages in life at every stage of the child's development.

Balance is knowing and teaching that everything functions in this world with a physical, mental, emotional and spiritual body and in order to be a whole person all of these faculties must be nurtured with care and commitment.

Righteousness involves teaching the children the laws of the creator, the laws of the land and their relationship with both so that their experiences are aligned with creative intention.

Harmony teaches the relationship of the creator and the created, the relationship between man and nature, and the relationship between man and fellow man and how each relationship is interdependent and necessary.

The polyandry family comes together with the wisdom that the nature of the creator is change. In order to manifest divine will, they must maintain consistency. Their reconnection in this most divine manner should be spoken to the world through ritual and ceremony put forth by our ancestors to allow the world to witness their commitment to oneness.

Marriage and Family Counseling with an unbiased spiritual counselor is highly recommended before any commitments in polyandry are made.

POLYAMORY as a stable family structure which include, more than one woman and more than one man. Each member of the family openly share their gifts to facilitate balance in the everyday quest of fulfilling each members divine purpose. They live as male and female couples and create a life of harmony that allows for spiritual, mental, emotional and financial success.

There is a recurring theme here that I want you to take note of: **spiritual discipline and purpose**. If this is not your intention in any relationship that you have, whether it be sexual or not, check yourself to be sure you are not spreading dysfunctional behavior and the pain it breeds. **Also, if you change your mind about the type of family structure you need for fulfilling your divine purpose, have the courage to communicate with your partner(s) to facilitate positive change.**

Once individuals can come together and operate with a free flowing level of commitment; then life can begin to be in alignment with a family's higher good.

Unfortunately, many who choose multi-family structures miss the most crucial necessity for a successful relationship of any kind, and that is you cannot enter into a spiritually correct union until you have yourself together! So if any person in the relationship is still carrying around levels and categories of dysfunctional ways like poor eating habits, social vices, emotional immaturity, negativity, hate for other people, lies and spiritual immaturity, then there will be problems that will facilitate consistent states of perpetual unhappiness. If you are already in a relationship or union and your mate(s) are currently dealing with these types of issues, then there needs to be some conversations on establishing a healing forum within your current union to help each other come out of these levels of dysfunction.

Help each other to become spiritually correct with each other. Spiritually correct unions have nothing to do with religion, it has everything to do with purpose living, unconditional care and commitment consistency. Living according to the dictates of the universe and divine law are beyond religion. However, if people would really practice their religions the way they should, then spiritual unions can be successful. Unfortunately, man has added so many of his idiosyncrasies into religion, and that too makes relationships dysfunctional.

Sex without relationship is missing a component of life energy that elevates the conscious mind. Therefore, holistic sexual living should be an attainable goal.

Chapter 6

The Next Generation

Teaching children about sex is a very delicate subject. Because it is a natural part of their basic instinct as children age, parents are often cautious of revealing certain aspects of sexuality to their children based on the fears that they carry about their own sexual lives. Parents sometimes instill those same fears in their children or even worse teach them nothing at all about their sexual nature. From a holistic point of view, it is better that a parent or elder who has the knowledge of holistic sexuality take the time to nurture the minds and hearts of the young ones on this subject.

Providing a system of security through knowledge and truth is the best method of sex education. There is no shame in security. The children should not be taught to hide their feelings and urges, instead they should learn to recognize them and bring them forth in family discussion when they appear, so that the proper acknowledgement of the growth that they are going through can be directed. Create a level of understanding and communication about sex that does not strike fear into the child about something that is as natural for them as breathing. Children love to talk and their experiences in life fuel their conversations. If children are taught to be afraid they will not learn affective communication. Instead they will learn to hide what they think others don't want to hear or they will shut down in silent suffering because they don't want the people in their lives, namely parents, to condemn them. There are grown people today who still cannot talk to their parents without the fear of ridicule.

Children become aware of their bodies, genitals and attractions as early as four years old. For parents and caretakers that observe this stage of development, it is necessary to have age appropriate information available to explain and guide the young ones to a place of balance in their growth process. Some of the topics that parents should be prepared to discuss are sexual anatomy, the differences between girls and boys, procreation, attraction to the opposite sex, what is appropriate and not appropriate for their age of development and the cycles of order that will require certain levels of responsibility to fulfill for growing up strong.

Puberty should be looked at as a celebration of life and growth. It is a rite of passage for young women and young men to enter the realm of adulthood. When children are taught to honor and respect procreation, they are more likely to make decisions in life that reflect their learning. If young men are taught to honor women, even if she does not know herself, there will be a lesser chance that these young men will act with disrespect toward any divine feminine. If young women are taught from an early age to honor and respect the divine masculine reflection of their male peers, this will allow the blending of righteousness and compromise to guide all their relationships with the young men they encounter.

Children should receive guidance on their first encounters of attraction. Often young people feel the draw of each other, however, once they have the knowledge of exactly what that attraction is, they are able to use their wisdom faculty to help them think about their actions and reactions to their feelings.

Children should also be taught about peer pressure and how to respond to these mental and emotional attacks from those who have not been trained in the ways of balance. If someone is worthy of their time, they will first align themselves with the family through a meeting to discuss their intentions. If the young man or the young woman cannot bring the person home that they are attracted to, there is either an imbalance in the family or an imbalance in their intentions. Remember, there is no shame in learning to grow in holistic sexuality.

However, the ways of the world have a great influence on the youth of today, no matter what conditions a family creates, there is still the possibility that they will receive information that contradicts the teachings of righteousness, and the youth may find themselves making decisions that are contrary to their upbringing. If this is one of the life lessons of your youth's journey, then as a parent of wisdom, it will required that you unconditionally accept their choices and give your support for the changes they will go through in life.

A major fear factor in teaching the youth about sex is the reality of teenage pregnancy. Because parents and care givers put so much of their expectations into what they think the future life of their children should hold, they often do not honor the beauty of procreation when their children make the decisions to explore their sexuality and the result is the life of a beautiful soul trying to come through their bloodline. All human life is sacred no matter the channels that it chooses to come through. When young people make the decision to explore their natural sexual desires and urges and a child is the result, parents and caregivers should offer supports that honors the value of all life.

Teaching the youth about sex is an area that can only be done by those that truly embrace a commitment to the truth about the human body without the societal hang-ups that promote dysfunctional sexual behavior.

Sex education in the form of family or community Rites of Passage is another way of ensuring balance if parents are not equipped or ready to offer a holistic way of learning about sex. Most communities are still in the process of developing programs and ceremonies that will bring honor to this growth process without shame. Check with your local culturally conscious community center for information on youth rites of passage programs.

Chapter 7

Holistic Sexual Living

When holistic sexuality becomes a part of the norm in life, you will use your sexual power to heal your mate(s) and enhance your lives together. You will use your sexual powers to manifest things in your life that are for the greater good of the family. Imagine being a force of positive energy that is renewable and everlasting.

Sex is that divine tool that has been given to assist people in reaching those higher levels of consciousness as it relates to the human physical, mental and emotional presence in this space and time. Holistic sexuality moves families out of dysfunctional ways of living and allows humans to relate together on a whole level of caring and sharing.

The bottom line is to manifest life the way the creator intended for it to be. You are procreating a holistic life mentally, spiritually, emotionally and spiritually when you change your thoughts and actions about sex. You are connecting to the divine.

Holistic sexual living is healing energy for your growth and progress. Once you decide to start using holistic sexuality, things are going to change automatically. You will begin to see old things fall away and new things come into being.

Holistic sexual living first requires honest communications. If honesty can be mastered where speaking the truth is a non issue, it will help calm the immature emotional responses that couples often have to work through. The greatest emotional hindrance to living a holistic sexual lifestyle is mastering non-possessive behavior, eliminate this and life will flourish with healing energy. The healing energy of life gets you through the physical, mental, emotional and spiritual transitions as you grow as a family and it keeps everyone in sync with the natural rhythms of being divine masculine and divine feminine.

Spiritually correct unions, no matter which family structure is chosen, should promote the growth and progress of each family member. This unconditional support solidifies the connection to the divine.

Bibliography

Afua, Queen (2010) *Overcoming An Angry Vagina*. New York, NY: Black Anhk Publications

Ammi, Ben (2010) *Physical Immortality Conquering Death*. Dimona, Israel: Communicators Press

Ashby, Muata (2006) *Egyptian Tantric Yoga*. Miami, FL: Cruzian Mystic Books

Gray, K. Akua (2013) *Natural Health and Wellness Manual*. Missouri City, TX: Bojakaz Management

Jaha, Niambi (2008) *Project Butterfly*. Perfect Books

Sherwood, Keith (2002) *Chakra Therapy* . Woodbury, MN: Llewellyn Publications